This Book Belongs To:

NAME: ____________________

EMERGENCY CONTACT: ____________________

EMERGENCY CONTACT: ____________________

GENERIC NAME:	DRUG NAME:
DRUG CLASS:	HIGH ALERT STATUS: YES: ☐ NO: ☐

MECHANISMS OF ACTION:	CONTRAINDICATIONS:	SAFETY & ANTIDOTE:
DOSAGE & ROUTE:	SIDE EFFECTS: (ADVERSE REACTION)	THERAPEUPIC USE:

PATIENT EDUCATION:	NURSING ASSESSMENTS / INTERVENTIONS:

NOTE:

GENERIC NAME:	DRUG NAME:
DRUG CLASS:	HIGH ALERT STATUS: ☐ YES: ☐ NO:

MECHANISMS OF ACTION:	CONTRAINDICATIONS:	SAFETY & ANTIDOTE:
DOSAGE & ROUTE:	SIDE EFFECTS: (ADVERSE REACTION)	THERAPEUPIC USE:

PATIENT EDUCATION:	NURSING ASSESSMENTS / INTERVENTIONS:

NOTE:

GENERIC NAME:	DRUG NAME:
DRUG CLASS:	HIGH ALERT STATUS: ☐ YES: ☐ NO:

MECHANISMS OF ACTION:	CONTRAINDICATIONS:	SAFETY & ANTIDOTE:
DOSAGE & ROUTE:	SIDE EFFECTS: (ADVERSE REACTION)	THERAPEUPIC USE:

PATIENT EDUCATION:	NURSING ASSESSMENTS / INTERVENTIONS:

NOTE:

GENERIC NAME:	DRUG NAME:
DRUG CLASS:	HIGH ALERT STATUS: ☐ YES: ☐ NO:

MECHANISMS OF ACTION:	CONTRAINDICATIONS:	SAFETY & ANTIDOTE:
DOSAGE & ROUTE:	SIDE EFFECTS: (ADVERSE REACTION)	THERAPEUPIC USE:

PATIENT EDUCATION:	NURSING ASSESSMENTS / INTERVENTIONS:

NOTE:

GENERIC NAME:	DRUG NAME:
DRUG CLASS:	HIGH ALERT STATUS: ☐ YES: ☐ NO:

MECHANISMS OF ACTION:	CONTRAINDICATIONS:	SAFETY & ANTIDOTE:
DOSAGE & ROUTE:	SIDE EFFECTS: (ADVERSE REACTION)	THERAPEUPIC USE:

PATIENT EDUCATION:	NURSING ASSESSMENTS / INTERVENTIONS:

NOTE:

GENERIC NAME:	DRUG NAME:
DRUG CLASS:	HIGH ALERT STATUS: ☐ YES: ☐ NO:

MECHANISMS OF ACTION:	CONTRAINDICATIONS:	SAFETY & ANTIDOTE:
DOSAGE & ROUTE:	SIDE EFFECTS: (ADVERSE REACTION)	THERAPEUPIC USE:

PATIENT EDUCATION:	NURSING ASSESSMENTS / INTERVENTIONS:

NOTE:

GENERIC NAME:	DRUG NAME:
DRUG CLASS:	HIGH ALERT STATUS: ☐ YES: ☐ NO:

MECHANISMS OF ACTION:	CONTRAINDICATIONS:	SAFETY & ANTIDOTE:
DOSAGE & ROUTE:	SIDE EFFECTS: (ADVERSE REACTION)	THERAPEUPIC USE:

PATIENT EDUCATION:	NURSING ASSESSMENTS / INTERVENTIONS:

NOTE:

GENERIC NAME:	DRUG NAME:
DRUG CLASS:	HIGH ALERT STATUS: ☐ YES: ☐ NO:

MECHANISMS OF ACTION:	CONTRAINDICATIONS:	SAFETY & ANTIDOTE:
DOSAGE & ROUTE:	SIDE EFFECTS: (ADVERSE REACTION)	THERAPEUPIC USE:

PATIENT EDUCATION:	NURSING ASSESSMENTS / INTERVENTIONS:

NOTE:

GENERIC NAME:	DRUG NAME:
DRUG CLASS:	HIGH ALERT STATUS: ☐ YES: ☐ NO:

MECHANISMS OF ACTION:	CONTRAINDICATIONS:	SAFETY & ANTIDOTE:
DOSAGE & ROUTE:	SIDE EFFECTS: (ADVERSE REACTION)	THERAPEUPIC USE:

PATIENT EDUCATION:	NURSING ASSESSMENTS / INTERVENTIONS:

NOTE:

GENERIC NAME:	**DRUG NAME:**
DRUG CLASS:	**HIGH ALERT STATUS:** ☐ YES: ☐ NO:

MECHANISMS OF ACTION:	**CONTRAINDICATIONS:**	**SAFETY & ANTIDOTE:**
DOSAGE & ROUTE:	**SIDE EFFECTS:** (ADVERSE REACTION)	**THERAPEUPIC USE:**

PATIENT EDUCATION:	**NURSING ASSESSMENTS / INTERVENTIONS:**

NOTE:

GENERIC NAME:	DRUG NAME:
DRUG CLASS:	HIGH ALERT STATUS: ☐ YES: ☐ NO:

MECHANISMS OF ACTION:	CONTRAINDICATIONS:	SAFETY & ANTIDOTE:
DOSAGE & ROUTE:	SIDE EFFECTS: (ADVERSE REACTION)	THERAPEUPIC USE:

PATIENT EDUCATION:	NURSING ASSESSMENTS / INTERVENTIONS:

NOTE:

GENERIC NAME:	DRUG NAME:
DRUG CLASS:	HIGH ALERT STATUS: ☐ YES: ☐ NO:

MECHANISMS OF ACTION:	CONTRAINDICATIONS:	SAFETY & ANTIDOTE:
DOSAGE & ROUTE:	SIDE EFFECTS: (ADVERSE REACTION)	THERAPEUPIC USE:

PATIENT EDUCATION:	NURSING ASSESSMENTS / INTERVENTIONS:

NOTE:

GENERIC NAME:	DRUG NAME:
DRUG CLASS:	HIGH ALERT STATUS: ☐ YES: ☐ NO:

MECHANISMS OF ACTION:	CONTRAINDICATIONS:	SAFETY & ANTIDOTE:
DOSAGE & ROUTE:	SIDE EFFECTS: (ADVERSE REACTION)	THERAPEUPIC USE:

PATIENT EDUCATION:	NURSING ASSESSMENTS / INTERVENTIONS:

NOTE:

GENERIC NAME:	DRUG NAME:
DRUG CLASS:	HIGH ALERT STATUS: ☐ YES: ☐ NO:

MECHANISMS OF ACTION:	CONTRAINDICATIONS:	SAFETY & ANTIDOTE:
DOSAGE & ROUTE:	SIDE EFFECTS: (ADVERSE REACTION)	THERAPEUPIC USE:

PATIENT EDUCATION:	NURSING ASSESSMENTS / INTERVENTIONS:

NOTE:

GENERIC NAME:	DRUG NAME:
DRUG CLASS:	HIGH ALERT STATUS: ☐ YES: ☐ NO:

MECHANISMS OF ACTION:	CONTRAINDICATIONS:	SAFETY & ANTIDOTE:
DOSAGE & ROUTE:	SIDE EFFECTS: (ADVERSE REACTION)	THERAPEUPIC USE:

PATIENT EDUCATION:	NURSING ASSESSMENTS / INTERVENTIONS:

NOTE:

GENERIC NAME:	DRUG NAME:
DRUG CLASS:	HIGH ALERT STATUS: ☐ YES: ☐ NO:

MECHANISMS OF ACTION:	CONTRAINDICATIONS:	SAFETY & ANTIDOTE:
DOSAGE & ROUTE:	SIDE EFFECTS: (ADVERSE REACTION)	THERAPEUPIC USE:

PATIENT EDUCATION:	NURSING ASSESSMENTS / INTERVENTIONS:

NOTE:

GENERIC NAME:	DRUG NAME:
DRUG CLASS:	HIGH ALERT STATUS: ☐ YES: ☐ NO:

MECHANISMS OF ACTION:	CONTRAINDICATIONS:	SAFETY & ANTIDOTE:
DOSAGE & ROUTE:	SIDE EFFECTS: (ADVERSE REACTION)	THERAPEUPIC USE:

PATIENT EDUCATION:	NURSING ASSESSMENTS / INTERVENTIONS:

NOTE:

GENERIC NAME:	DRUG NAME:
DRUG CLASS:	HIGH ALERT STATUS: ☐ YES: ☐ NO:

MECHANISMS OF ACTION:	CONTRAINDICATIONS:	SAFETY & ANTIDOTE:
DOSAGE & ROUTE:	SIDE EFFECTS: (ADVERSE REACTION)	THERAPEUPIC USE:

PATIENT EDUCATION:	NURSING ASSESSMENTS / INTERVENTIONS:

NOTE:

GENERIC NAME:	DRUG NAME:
DRUG CLASS:	HIGH ALERT STATUS: ☐ YES: ☐ NO:

MECHANISMS OF ACTION:	CONTRAINDICATIONS:	SAFETY & ANTIDOTE:
DOSAGE & ROUTE:	SIDE EFFECTS: (ADVERSE REACTION)	THERAPEUPIC USE:

PATIENT EDUCATION:	NURSING ASSESSMENTS / INTERVENTIONS:

NOTE:

GENERIC NAME:	DRUG NAME:
DRUG CLASS:	HIGH ALERT STATUS: ☐ YES: ☐ NO:

MECHANISMS OF ACTION:	CONTRAINDICATIONS:	SAFETY & ANTIDOTE:
DOSAGE & ROUTE:	SIDE EFFECTS: (ADVERSE REACTION)	THERAPEUPIC USE:

PATIENT EDUCATION:	NURSING ASSESSMENTS / INTERVENTIONS:

NOTE:

GENERIC NAME:	**DRUG NAME:**
DRUG CLASS:	**HIGH ALERT STATUS:** ☐ YES: ☐ NO:

MECHANISMS OF ACTION:	**CONTRAINDICATIONS:**	**SAFETY & ANTIDOTE:**
DOSAGE & ROUTE:	**SIDE EFFECTS:** (ADVERSE REACTION)	**THERAPEUPIC USE:**

PATIENT EDUCATION:	**NURSING ASSESSMENTS / INTERVENTIONS:**

NOTE:

GENERIC NAME:	DRUG NAME:
DRUG CLASS:	HIGH ALERT STATUS: ☐ YES: ☐ NO:

MECHANISMS OF ACTION:	CONTRAINDICATIONS:	SAFETY & ANTIDOTE:
DOSAGE & ROUTE:	SIDE EFFECTS: (ADVERSE REACTION)	THERAPEUPIC USE:

PATIENT EDUCATION:	NURSING ASSESSMENTS / INTERVENTIONS:

NOTE:

GENERIC NAME:	DRUG NAME:
DRUG CLASS:	HIGH ALERT STATUS: ☐ YES: ☐ NO:

MECHANISMS OF ACTION:	CONTRAINDICATIONS:	SAFETY & ANTIDOTE:
DOSAGE & ROUTE:	SIDE EFFECTS: (ADVERSE REACTION)	THERAPEUPIC USE:

PATIENT EDUCATION:	NURSING ASSESSMENTS / INTERVENTIONS:

NOTE:

GENERIC NAME:	DRUG NAME:
DRUG CLASS:	HIGH ALERT STATUS: ☐ YES: ☐ NO:

MECHANISMS OF ACTION:	CONTRAINDICATIONS:	SAFETY & ANTIDOTE:
DOSAGE & ROUTE:	SIDE EFFECTS: (ADVERSE REACTION)	THERAPEUPIC USE:

PATIENT EDUCATION:	NURSING ASSESSMENTS / INTERVENTIONS:

NOTE:

GENERIC NAME:	DRUG NAME:
DRUG CLASS:	HIGH ALERT STATUS: ☐ YES: ☐ NO:

MECHANISMS OF ACTION:	CONTRAINDICATIONS:	SAFETY & ANTIDOTE:
DOSAGE & ROUTE:	SIDE EFFECTS: (ADVERSE REACTION)	THERAPEUPIC USE:

PATIENT EDUCATION:	NURSING ASSESSMENTS / INTERVENTIONS:

NOTE:

GENERIC NAME:	DRUG NAME:
DRUG CLASS:	HIGH ALERT STATUS: ☐ YES: ☐ NO:

MECHANISMS OF ACTION:	CONTRAINDICATIONS:	SAFETY & ANTIDOTE:
DOSAGE & ROUTE:	SIDE EFFECTS: (ADVERSE REACTION)	THERAPEUPIC USE:

PATIENT EDUCATION:	NURSING ASSESSMENTS / INTERVENTIONS:

NOTE:

GENERIC NAME:	DRUG NAME:
DRUG CLASS:	HIGH ALERT STATUS: ☐ YES: ☐ NO:

MECHANISMS OF ACTION:	CONTRAINDICATIONS:	SAFETY & ANTIDOTE:
DOSAGE & ROUTE:	SIDE EFFECTS: (ADVERSE REACTION)	THERAPEUPIC USE:

PATIENT EDUCATION:	NURSING ASSESSMENTS / INTERVENTIONS:

NOTE:

GENERIC NAME:

DRUG NAME:

DRUG CLASS:

HIGH ALERT STATUS: ☐ YES: ☐ NO:

MECHANISMS OF ACTION:

CONTRAINDICATIONS:

SAFETY & ANTIDOTE:

DOSAGE & ROUTE:

SIDE EFFECTS:
(ADVERSE REACTION)

THERAPEUPIC USE:

PATIENT EDUCATION:

NURSING ASSESSMENTS / INTERVENTIONS:

NOTE:

GENERIC NAME:	DRUG NAME:
DRUG CLASS:	HIGH ALERT STATUS: ☐ YES: ☐ NO:

MECHANISMS OF ACTION:	CONTRAINDICATIONS:	SAFETY & ANTIDOTE:
DOSAGE & ROUTE:	SIDE EFFECTS: (ADVERSE REACTION)	THERAPEUPIC USE:

PATIENT EDUCATION:	NURSING ASSESSMENTS / INTERVENTIONS:

NOTE:

GENERIC NAME:	DRUG NAME:
DRUG CLASS:	HIGH ALERT STATUS: ☐ YES: ☐ NO:

MECHANISMS OF ACTION:	CONTRAINDICATIONS:	SAFETY & ANTIDOTE:
DOSAGE & ROUTE:	SIDE EFFECTS: (ADVERSE REACTION)	THERAPEUPIC USE:

PATIENT EDUCATION:	NURSING ASSESSMENTS / INTERVENTIONS:

NOTE:

GENERIC NAME:	DRUG NAME:
DRUG CLASS:	HIGH ALERT STATUS: ☐ YES: ☐ NO:

MECHANISMS OF ACTION:	CONTRAINDICATIONS:	SAFETY & ANTIDOTE:
DOSAGE & ROUTE:	SIDE EFFECTS: (ADVERSE REACTION)	THERAPEUPIC USE:

PATIENT EDUCATION:	NURSING ASSESSMENTS / INTERVENTIONS:

NOTE:

GENERIC NAME:	DRUG NAME:
DRUG CLASS:	HIGH ALERT STATUS: ☐ YES: ☐ NO:

MECHANISMS OF ACTION:	CONTRAINDICATIONS:	SAFETY & ANTIDOTE:
DOSAGE & ROUTE:	SIDE EFFECTS: (ADVERSE REACTION)	THERAPEUPIC USE:

PATIENT EDUCATION:	NURSING ASSESSMENTS / INTERVENTIONS:

NOTE:

GENERIC NAME:	DRUG NAME:
DRUG CLASS:	HIGH ALERT STATUS: ☐ YES: ☐ NO:

MECHANISMS OF ACTION:	CONTRAINDICATIONS:	SAFETY & ANTIDOTE:
DOSAGE & ROUTE:	SIDE EFFECTS: (ADVERSE REACTION)	THERAPEUPIC USE:

PATIENT EDUCATION:	NURSING ASSESSMENTS / INTERVENTIONS:

NOTE:

GENERIC NAME:	DRUG NAME:
DRUG CLASS:	HIGH ALERT STATUS: ☐ YES: ☐ NO:

MECHANISMS OF ACTION:	CONTRAINDICATIONS:	SAFETY & ANTIDOTE:
DOSAGE & ROUTE:	SIDE EFFECTS: (ADVERSE REACTION)	THERAPEUPIC USE:

PATIENT EDUCATION:	NURSING ASSESSMENTS / INTERVENTIONS:

NOTE:

GENERIC NAME:	**DRUG NAME:**
DRUG CLASS:	**HIGH ALERT STATUS:** ☐ YES: ☐ NO:

MECHANISMS OF ACTION:	**CONTRAINDICATIONS:**	**SAFETY & ANTIDOTE:**
DOSAGE & ROUTE:	**SIDE EFFECTS:** (ADVERSE REACTION)	**THERAPEUPIC USE:**

PATIENT EDUCATION:	**NURSING ASSESSMENTS / INTERVENTIONS:**

NOTE:

GENERIC NAME:	DRUG NAME:
DRUG CLASS:	HIGH ALERT STATUS: ☐ YES: ☐ NO:

MECHANISMS OF ACTION:	CONTRAINDICATIONS:	SAFETY & ANTIDOTE:
DOSAGE & ROUTE:	SIDE EFFECTS: (ADVERSE REACTION)	THERAPEUPIC USE:

PATIENT EDUCATION:	NURSING ASSESSMENTS / INTERVENTIONS:

NOTE:

GENERIC NAME:	DRUG NAME:
DRUG CLASS:	HIGH ALERT STATUS: ☐ YES: ☐ NO:

MECHANISMS OF ACTION:	CONTRAINDICATIONS:	SAFETY & ANTIDOTE:
DOSAGE & ROUTE:	SIDE EFFECTS: (ADVERSE REACTION)	THERAPEUPIC USE:

PATIENT EDUCATION:	NURSING ASSESSMENTS / INTERVENTIONS:

NOTE:

GENERIC NAME:	DRUG NAME:
DRUG CLASS:	HIGH ALERT STATUS: ☐ YES: ☐ NO:

MECHANISMS OF ACTION:	CONTRAINDICATIONS:	SAFETY & ANTIDOTE:
DOSAGE & ROUTE:	SIDE EFFECTS: (ADVERSE REACTION)	THERAPEUPIC USE:

PATIENT EDUCATION:	NURSING ASSESSMENTS / INTERVENTIONS:

NOTE:

GENERIC NAME:	DRUG NAME:
DRUG CLASS:	HIGH ALERT STATUS: YES: ☐ NO: ☐

MECHANISMS OF ACTION:	CONTRAINDICATIONS:	SAFETY & ANTIDOTE:
DOSAGE & ROUTE:	SIDE EFFECTS: (ADVERSE REACTION)	THERAPEUPIC USE:

PATIENT EDUCATION:	NURSING ASSESSMENTS / INTERVENTIONS:

NOTE:

GENERIC NAME:	DRUG NAME:
DRUG CLASS:	HIGH ALERT STATUS: ☐ YES: ☐ NO:

MECHANISMS OF ACTION:	CONTRAINDICATIONS:	SAFETY & ANTIDOTE:
DOSAGE & ROUTE:	SIDE EFFECTS: (ADVERSE REACTION)	THERAPEUPIC USE:

PATIENT EDUCATION:	NURSING ASSESSMENTS / INTERVENTIONS:

NOTE:

GENERIC NAME:	DRUG NAME:
DRUG CLASS:	HIGH ALERT STATUS: ☐ YES: ☐ NO:

MECHANISMS OF ACTION:	CONTRAINDICATIONS:	SAFETY & ANTIDOTE:
DOSAGE & ROUTE:	SIDE EFFECTS: (ADVERSE REACTION)	THERAPEUPIC USE:

PATIENT EDUCATION:	NURSING ASSESSMENTS / INTERVENTIONS:

NOTE:

GENERIC NAME:	DRUG NAME:
DRUG CLASS:	HIGH ALERT STATUS: ☐ YES: ☐ NO:

MECHANISMS OF ACTION:	CONTRAINDICATIONS:	SAFETY & ANTIDOTE:
DOSAGE & ROUTE:	SIDE EFFECTS: (ADVERSE REACTION)	THERAPEUPIC USE:

PATIENT EDUCATION:	NURSING ASSESSMENTS / INTERVENTIONS:

NOTE:

GENERIC NAME:

DRUG NAME:

DRUG CLASS:

HIGH ALERT STATUS: YES: NO:

MECHANISMS OF ACTION:

CONTRAINDICATIONS:

SAFETY & ANTIDOTE:

DOSAGE & ROUTE:

SIDE EFFECTS:
(ADVERSE REACTION)

THERAPEUPIC USE:

PATIENT EDUCATION:

NURSING ASSESSMENTS / INTERVENTIONS:

NOTE:

GENERIC NAME:	DRUG NAME:
DRUG CLASS:	HIGH ALERT STATUS: ☐ YES: ☐ NO:

MECHANISMS OF ACTION:	CONTRAINDICATIONS:	SAFETY & ANTIDOTE:
DOSAGE & ROUTE:	SIDE EFFECTS: (ADVERSE REACTION)	THERAPEUPIC USE:

PATIENT EDUCATION:	NURSING ASSESSMENTS / INTERVENTIONS:

NOTE:

GENERIC NAME:	DRUG NAME:
DRUG CLASS:	HIGH ALERT STATUS: YES: ☐ NO: ☐

MECHANISMS OF ACTION:	CONTRAINDICATIONS:	SAFETY & ANTIDOTE:
DOSAGE & ROUTE:	SIDE EFFECTS: (ADVERSE REACTION)	THERAPEUPIC USE:

PATIENT EDUCATION:	NURSING ASSESSMENTS / INTERVENTIONS:

NOTE:

GENERIC NAME:	DRUG NAME:
DRUG CLASS:	HIGH ALERT STATUS: ☐ YES: ☐ NO:

MECHANISMS OF ACTION:	CONTRAINDICATIONS:	SAFETY & ANTIDOTE:
DOSAGE & ROUTE:	SIDE EFFECTS: (ADVERSE REACTION)	THERAPEUPIC USE:

PATIENT EDUCATION:	NURSING ASSESSMENTS / INTERVENTIONS:

NOTE:

GENERIC NAME:	DRUG NAME:
DRUG CLASS:	HIGH ALERT STATUS: ☐ YES: ☐ NO:

MECHANISMS OF ACTION:	CONTRAINDICATIONS:	SAFETY & ANTIDOTE:
DOSAGE & ROUTE:	SIDE EFFECTS: (ADVERSE REACTION)	THERAPEUPIC USE:

PATIENT EDUCATION:	NURSING ASSESSMENTS / INTERVENTIONS:

NOTE:

GENERIC NAME:	DRUG NAME:
DRUG CLASS:	HIGH ALERT STATUS: ☐ YES: ☐ NO:

MECHANISMS OF ACTION:	CONTRAINDICATIONS:	SAFETY & ANTIDOTE:
DOSAGE & ROUTE:	SIDE EFFECTS: (ADVERSE REACTION)	THERAPEUPIC USE:

PATIENT EDUCATION:	NURSING ASSESSMENTS / INTERVENTIONS:

NOTE:

GENERIC NAME:	DRUG NAME:
DRUG CLASS:	HIGH ALERT STATUS: ☐ YES: ☐ NO:

MECHANISMS OF ACTION:	CONTRAINDICATIONS:	SAFETY & ANTIDOTE:
DOSAGE & ROUTE:	SIDE EFFECTS: (ADVERSE REACTION)	THERAPEUPIC USE:

PATIENT EDUCATION:	NURSING ASSESSMENTS / INTERVENTIONS:

NOTE:

GENERIC NAME:	DRUG NAME:
DRUG CLASS:	HIGH ALERT STATUS: ☐ YES: ☐ NO:

MECHANISMS OF ACTION:	CONTRAINDICATIONS:	SAFETY & ANTIDOTE:
DOSAGE & ROUTE:	SIDE EFFECTS: (ADVERSE REACTION)	THERAPEUPIC USE:

PATIENT EDUCATION:	NURSING ASSESSMENTS / INTERVENTIONS:

NOTE:

GENERIC NAME:	DRUG NAME:
DRUG CLASS:	HIGH ALERT STATUS: ☐ YES: ☐ NO:

MECHANISMS OF ACTION:	CONTRAINDICATIONS:	SAFETY & ANTIDOTE:
DOSAGE & ROUTE:	SIDE EFFECTS: (ADVERSE REACTION)	THERAPEUPIC USE:

PATIENT EDUCATION:	NURSING ASSESSMENTS / INTERVENTIONS:

NOTE:

GENERIC NAME:	DRUG NAME:
DRUG CLASS:	HIGH ALERT STATUS: ☐ YES: ☐ NO:

MECHANISMS OF ACTION:	CONTRAINDICATIONS:	SAFETY & ANTIDOTE:
DOSAGE & ROUTE:	SIDE EFFECTS: (ADVERSE REACTION)	THERAPEUPIC USE:

PATIENT EDUCATION:	NURSING ASSESSMENTS / INTERVENTIONS:

NOTE:

GENERIC NAME:	DRUG NAME:
DRUG CLASS:	HIGH ALERT STATUS: ☐ YES: ☐ NO:

MECHANISMS OF ACTION:	CONTRAINDICATIONS:	SAFETY & ANTIDOTE:
DOSAGE & ROUTE:	SIDE EFFECTS: (ADVERSE REACTION)	THERAPEUPIC USE:

PATIENT EDUCATION:	NURSING ASSESSMENTS / INTERVENTIONS:

NOTE:

GENERIC NAME:	DRUG NAME:
DRUG CLASS:	HIGH ALERT STATUS: ☐ YES: ☐ NO:

MECHANISMS OF ACTION:	CONTRAINDICATIONS:	SAFETY & ANTIDOTE:
DOSAGE & ROUTE:	SIDE EFFECTS: (ADVERSE REACTION)	THERAPEUPIC USE:

PATIENT EDUCATION:	NURSING ASSESSMENTS / INTERVENTIONS:

NOTE:

GENERIC NAME:	DRUG NAME:
DRUG CLASS:	HIGH ALERT STATUS: ☐ YES: ☐ NO:

MECHANISMS OF ACTION:	CONTRAINDICATIONS:	SAFETY & ANTIDOTE:
DOSAGE & ROUTE:	SIDE EFFECTS: (ADVERSE REACTION)	THERAPEUPIC USE:

PATIENT EDUCATION:	NURSING ASSESSMENTS / INTERVENTIONS:

NOTE:

GENERIC NAME:	DRUG NAME:
DRUG CLASS:	HIGH ALERT STATUS: ☐ YES: ☐ NO:

MECHANISMS OF ACTION:	CONTRAINDICATIONS:	SAFETY & ANTIDOTE:
DOSAGE & ROUTE:	SIDE EFFECTS: (ADVERSE REACTION)	THERAPEUPIC USE:

PATIENT EDUCATION:	NURSING ASSESSMENTS / INTERVENTIONS:

NOTE:

GENERIC NAME:

DRUG NAME:

DRUG CLASS:

HIGH ALERT STATUS: YES: ☐ NO: ☐

MECHANISMS OF ACTION:

CONTRAINDICATIONS:

SAFETY & ANTIDOTE:

DOSAGE & ROUTE:

SIDE EFFECTS:
(ADVERSE REACTION)

THERAPEUPIC USE:

PATIENT EDUCATION:

NURSING ASSESSMENTS / INTERVENTIONS:

NOTE:

GENERIC NAME:	DRUG NAME:
DRUG CLASS:	HIGH ALERT STATUS: ☐ YES: ☐ NO:

MECHANISMS OF ACTION:	CONTRAINDICATIONS:	SAFETY & ANTIDOTE:
DOSAGE & ROUTE:	SIDE EFFECTS: (ADVERSE REACTION)	THERAPEUPIC USE:

PATIENT EDUCATION:	NURSING ASSESSMENTS / INTERVENTIONS:

NOTE:

GENERIC NAME:	DRUG NAME:
DRUG CLASS:	HIGH ALERT STATUS: ☐ YES: ☐ NO:

MECHANISMS OF ACTION:	CONTRAINDICATIONS:	SAFETY & ANTIDOTE:
DOSAGE & ROUTE:	SIDE EFFECTS: (ADVERSE REACTION)	THERAPEUPIC USE:

PATIENT EDUCATION:	NURSING ASSESSMENTS / INTERVENTIONS:

NOTE:

GENERIC NAME:	DRUG NAME:
DRUG CLASS:	HIGH ALERT STATUS: ☐ YES: ☐ NO:

MECHANISMS OF ACTION:	CONTRAINDICATIONS:	SAFETY & ANTIDOTE:
DOSAGE & ROUTE:	SIDE EFFECTS: (ADVERSE REACTION)	THERAPEUPIC USE:

PATIENT EDUCATION:	NURSING ASSESSMENTS / INTERVENTIONS:

NOTE:

GENERIC NAME:	DRUG NAME:
DRUG CLASS:	HIGH ALERT STATUS: ☐ YES: ☐ NO:

MECHANISMS OF ACTION:	CONTRAINDICATIONS:	SAFETY & ANTIDOTE:
DOSAGE & ROUTE:	SIDE EFFECTS: (ADVERSE REACTION)	THERAPEUPIC USE:

PATIENT EDUCATION:	NURSING ASSESSMENTS / INTERVENTIONS:

NOTE:

GENERIC NAME:	DRUG NAME:
DRUG CLASS:	HIGH ALERT STATUS: ☐ YES: ☐ NO:

MECHANISMS OF ACTION:	CONTRAINDICATIONS:	SAFETY & ANTIDOTE:
DOSAGE & ROUTE:	SIDE EFFECTS: (ADVERSE REACTION)	THERAPEUPIC USE:

PATIENT EDUCATION:	NURSING ASSESSMENTS / INTERVENTIONS:

NOTE:

GENERIC NAME:	DRUG NAME:
DRUG CLASS:	HIGH ALERT STATUS: ☐ YES: ☐ NO:

MECHANISMS OF ACTION:	CONTRAINDICATIONS:	SAFETY & ANTIDOTE:
DOSAGE & ROUTE:	SIDE EFFECTS: (ADVERSE REACTION)	THERAPEUPIC USE:

PATIENT EDUCATION:	NURSING ASSESSMENTS / INTERVENTIONS:

NOTE:

GENERIC NAME:	DRUG NAME:
DRUG CLASS:	HIGH ALERT STATUS: ☐ YES: ☐ NO:

MECHANISMS OF ACTION:	CONTRAINDICATIONS:	SAFETY & ANTIDOTE:
DOSAGE & ROUTE:	SIDE EFFECTS: (ADVERSE REACTION)	THERAPEUPIC USE:

PATIENT EDUCATION:	NURSING ASSESSMENTS / INTERVENTIONS:

NOTE:

GENERIC NAME:	DRUG NAME:
DRUG CLASS:	HIGH ALERT STATUS: ☐ YES: ☐ NO:

MECHANISMS OF ACTION:	CONTRAINDICATIONS:	SAFETY & ANTIDOTE:
DOSAGE & ROUTE:	SIDE EFFECTS: (ADVERSE REACTION)	THERAPEUPIC USE:

PATIENT EDUCATION:	NURSING ASSESSMENTS / INTERVENTIONS:

NOTE:

GENERIC NAME:	DRUG NAME:
DRUG CLASS:	HIGH ALERT STATUS: ☐ YES: ☐ NO:

MECHANISMS OF ACTION:	CONTRAINDICATIONS:	SAFETY & ANTIDOTE:
DOSAGE & ROUTE:	SIDE EFFECTS: (ADVERSE REACTION)	THERAPEUPIC USE:

PATIENT EDUCATION:	NURSING ASSESSMENTS / INTERVENTIONS:

NOTE:

GENERIC NAME:	**DRUG NAME:**
DRUG CLASS:	**HIGH ALERT STATUS:** ☐ YES: ☐ NO:

MECHANISMS OF ACTION:	**CONTRAINDICATIONS:**	**SAFETY & ANTIDOTE:**
DOSAGE & ROUTE:	**SIDE EFFECTS:** (ADVERSE REACTION)	**THERAPEUPIC USE:**

PATIENT EDUCATION:	**NURSING ASSESSMENTS / INTERVENTIONS:**

NOTE:

GENERIC NAME:	DRUG NAME:
DRUG CLASS:	HIGH ALERT STATUS: ☐ YES: ☐ NO:

MECHANISMS OF ACTION:	CONTRAINDICATIONS:	SAFETY & ANTIDOTE:
DOSAGE & ROUTE:	SIDE EFFECTS: (ADVERSE REACTION)	THERAPEUPIC USE:

PATIENT EDUCATION:	NURSING ASSESSMENTS / INTERVENTIONS:

NOTE:

GENERIC NAME:	DRUG NAME:
DRUG CLASS:	HIGH ALERT STATUS: YES: [ ] NO: [ ]

MECHANISMS OF ACTION:	CONTRAINDICATIONS:	SAFETY & ANTIDOTE:
DOSAGE & ROUTE:	SIDE EFFECTS: (ADVERSE REACTION)	THERAPEUPIC USE:

PATIENT EDUCATION:	NURSING ASSESSMENTS / INTERVENTIONS:

NOTE:

GENERIC NAME:	DRUG NAME:
DRUG CLASS:	HIGH ALERT STATUS: ☐ YES: ☐ NO:

MECHANISMS OF ACTION:	CONTRAINDICATIONS:	SAFETY & ANTIDOTE:
DOSAGE & ROUTE:	SIDE EFFECTS: (ADVERSE REACTION)	THERAPEUPIC USE:

PATIENT EDUCATION:	NURSING ASSESSMENTS / INTERVENTIONS:

NOTE:

GENERIC NAME:	DRUG NAME:
DRUG CLASS:	HIGH ALERT STATUS: ☐ YES: ☐ NO:

MECHANISMS OF ACTION:	CONTRAINDICATIONS:	SAFETY & ANTIDOTE:
DOSAGE & ROUTE:	SIDE EFFECTS: (ADVERSE REACTION)	THERAPEUPIC USE:

PATIENT EDUCATION:	NURSING ASSESSMENTS / INTERVENTIONS:

NOTE:

GENERIC NAME:	DRUG NAME:
DRUG CLASS:	HIGH ALERT STATUS: ☐ YES: ☐ NO:

MECHANISMS OF ACTION:	CONTRAINDICATIONS:	SAFETY & ANTIDOTE:
DOSAGE & ROUTE:	SIDE EFFECTS: (ADVERSE REACTION)	THERAPEUPIC USE:

PATIENT EDUCATION:	NURSING ASSESSMENTS / INTERVENTIONS:

NOTE:

GENERIC NAME:	DRUG NAME:
DRUG CLASS:	HIGH ALERT STATUS: ☐ YES: ☐ NO:

MECHANISMS OF ACTION:	CONTRAINDICATIONS:	SAFETY & ANTIDOTE:
DOSAGE & ROUTE:	SIDE EFFECTS: (ADVERSE REACTION)	THERAPEUPIC USE:

PATIENT EDUCATION:	NURSING ASSESSMENTS / INTERVENTIONS:

NOTE:

GENERIC NAME:	DRUG NAME:
DRUG CLASS:	HIGH ALERT STATUS: ☐ YES: ☐ NO:

MECHANISMS OF ACTION:	CONTRAINDICATIONS:	SAFETY & ANTIDOTE:
DOSAGE & ROUTE:	SIDE EFFECTS: (ADVERSE REACTION)	THERAPEUPIC USE:

PATIENT EDUCATION:	NURSING ASSESSMENTS / INTERVENTIONS:

NOTE:

GENERIC NAME:	DRUG NAME:
DRUG CLASS:	HIGH ALERT STATUS: ☐ YES: ☐ NO:

MECHANISMS OF ACTION:	CONTRAINDICATIONS:	SAFETY & ANTIDOTE:
DOSAGE & ROUTE:	SIDE EFFECTS: (ADVERSE REACTION)	THERAPEUPIC USE:

PATIENT EDUCATION:	NURSING ASSESSMENTS / INTERVENTIONS:

NOTE:

GENERIC NAME:	DRUG NAME:
DRUG CLASS:	HIGH ALERT STATUS: ☐ YES: ☐ NO:

MECHANISMS OF ACTION:	CONTRAINDICATIONS:	SAFETY & ANTIDOTE:
DOSAGE & ROUTE:	SIDE EFFECTS: (ADVERSE REACTION)	THERAPEUPIC USE:

PATIENT EDUCATION:	NURSING ASSESSMENTS / INTERVENTIONS:

NOTE:

GENERIC NAME:	DRUG NAME:
DRUG CLASS:	HIGH ALERT STATUS: ☐ YES: ☐ NO:

MECHANISMS OF ACTION:	CONTRAINDICATIONS:	SAFETY & ANTIDOTE:
DOSAGE & ROUTE:	SIDE EFFECTS: (ADVERSE REACTION)	THERAPEUPIC USE:

PATIENT EDUCATION:	NURSING ASSESSMENTS / INTERVENTIONS:

NOTE:

GENERIC NAME:	DRUG NAME:
DRUG CLASS:	HIGH ALERT STATUS: ☐ YES: ☐ NO:

MECHANISMS OF ACTION:	CONTRAINDICATIONS:	SAFETY & ANTIDOTE:
DOSAGE & ROUTE:	SIDE EFFECTS: (ADVERSE REACTION)	THERAPEUPIC USE:

PATIENT EDUCATION:	NURSING ASSESSMENTS / INTERVENTIONS:

NOTE:

GENERIC NAME:	DRUG NAME:
DRUG CLASS:	HIGH ALERT STATUS: ☐ YES: ☐ NO:

MECHANISMS OF ACTION:	CONTRAINDICATIONS:	SAFETY & ANTIDOTE:
DOSAGE & ROUTE:	SIDE EFFECTS: (ADVERSE REACTION)	THERAPEUPIC USE:

PATIENT EDUCATION:	NURSING ASSESSMENTS / INTERVENTIONS:

NOTE:

GENERIC NAME:	DRUG NAME:
DRUG CLASS:	HIGH ALERT STATUS: ☐ YES: ☐ NO:

MECHANISMS OF ACTION:	CONTRAINDICATIONS:	SAFETY & ANTIDOTE:
DOSAGE & ROUTE:	SIDE EFFECTS: (ADVERSE REACTION)	THERAPEUPIC USE:

PATIENT EDUCATION:	NURSING ASSESSMENTS / INTERVENTIONS:

NOTE:

GENERIC NAME:	DRUG NAME:
DRUG CLASS:	HIGH ALERT STATUS: ☐ YES: ☐ NO:

MECHANISMS OF ACTION:	CONTRAINDICATIONS:	SAFETY & ANTIDOTE:
DOSAGE & ROUTE:	SIDE EFFECTS: (ADVERSE REACTION)	THERAPEUPIC USE:

PATIENT EDUCATION:	NURSING ASSESSMENTS / INTERVENTIONS:

NOTE:

GENERIC NAME:	DRUG NAME:
DRUG CLASS:	HIGH ALERT STATUS: ☐ YES: ☐ NO:

MECHANISMS OF ACTION:	CONTRAINDICATIONS:	SAFETY & ANTIDOTE:
DOSAGE & ROUTE:	SIDE EFFECTS: (ADVERSE REACTION)	THERAPEUPIC USE:

PATIENT EDUCATION:	NURSING ASSESSMENTS / INTERVENTIONS:

NOTE:

GENERIC NAME:	DRUG NAME:
DRUG CLASS:	HIGH ALERT STATUS: ☐ YES: ☐ NO:

MECHANISMS OF ACTION:	CONTRAINDICATIONS:	SAFETY & ANTIDOTE:
DOSAGE & ROUTE:	SIDE EFFECTS: (ADVERSE REACTION)	THERAPEUPIC USE:

PATIENT EDUCATION:	NURSING ASSESSMENTS / INTERVENTIONS:

NOTE:

GENERIC NAME:	DRUG NAME:
DRUG CLASS:	HIGH ALERT STATUS: ☐ YES: ☐ NO:

MECHANISMS OF ACTION:	CONTRAINDICATIONS:	SAFETY & ANTIDOTE:
DOSAGE & ROUTE:	SIDE EFFECTS: (ADVERSE REACTION)	THERAPEUPIC USE:

PATIENT EDUCATION:	NURSING ASSESSMENTS / INTERVENTIONS:

NOTE:

GENERIC NAME:	DRUG NAME:
DRUG CLASS:	HIGH ALERT STATUS: ☐ YES: ☐ NO:

MECHANISMS OF ACTION:	CONTRAINDICATIONS:	SAFETY & ANTIDOTE:
DOSAGE & ROUTE:	SIDE EFFECTS: (ADVERSE REACTION)	THERAPEUPIC USE:

PATIENT EDUCATION:	NURSING ASSESSMENTS / INTERVENTIONS:

NOTE:

GENERIC NAME:	DRUG NAME:
DRUG CLASS:	HIGH ALERT STATUS: ☐ YES: ☐ NO:

MECHANISMS OF ACTION:	CONTRAINDICATIONS:	SAFETY & ANTIDOTE:
DOSAGE & ROUTE:	SIDE EFFECTS: (ADVERSE REACTION)	THERAPEUPIC USE:

PATIENT EDUCATION:	NURSING ASSESSMENTS / INTERVENTIONS:

NOTE:

GENERIC NAME:	DRUG NAME:
DRUG CLASS:	HIGH ALERT STATUS: ☐ YES: ☐ NO:

MECHANISMS OF ACTION:	CONTRAINDICATIONS:	SAFETY & ANTIDOTE:
DOSAGE & ROUTE:	SIDE EFFECTS: (ADVERSE REACTION)	THERAPEUPIC USE:

PATIENT EDUCATION:	NURSING ASSESSMENTS / INTERVENTIONS:

NOTE:

GENERIC NAME:	DRUG NAME:
DRUG CLASS:	HIGH ALERT STATUS: ☐ YES: ☐ NO:

MECHANISMS OF ACTION:	CONTRAINDICATIONS:	SAFETY & ANTIDOTE:
DOSAGE & ROUTE:	SIDE EFFECTS: (ADVERSE REACTION)	THERAPEUPIC USE:

PATIENT EDUCATION:	NURSING ASSESSMENTS / INTERVENTIONS:

NOTE:

GENERIC NAME:	**DRUG NAME:**
DRUG CLASS:	**HIGH ALERT STATUS:** ☐ YES: ☐ NO:

MECHANISMS OF ACTION:	**CONTRAINDICATIONS:**	**SAFETY & ANTIDOTE:**
DOSAGE & ROUTE:	**SIDE EFFECTS:** (ADVERSE REACTION)	**THERAPEUPIC USE:**

PATIENT EDUCATION:	**NURSING ASSESSMENTS / INTERVENTIONS:**

NOTE:

GENERIC NAME:	DRUG NAME:
DRUG CLASS:	HIGH ALERT STATUS: ☐ YES: ☐ NO:

MECHANISMS OF ACTION:	CONTRAINDICATIONS:	SAFETY & ANTIDOTE:
DOSAGE & ROUTE:	SIDE EFFECTS: (ADVERSE REACTION)	THERAPEUPIC USE:

PATIENT EDUCATION:	NURSING ASSESSMENTS / INTERVENTIONS:

NOTE:

GENERIC NAME:	DRUG NAME:
DRUG CLASS:	HIGH ALERT STATUS: ☐ YES: ☐ NO:

MECHANISMS OF ACTION:	CONTRAINDICATIONS:	SAFETY & ANTIDOTE:
DOSAGE & ROUTE:	SIDE EFFECTS: (ADVERSE REACTION)	THERAPEUPIC USE:

PATIENT EDUCATION:	NURSING ASSESSMENTS / INTERVENTIONS:

NOTE:

GENERIC NAME:	DRUG NAME:
DRUG CLASS:	HIGH ALERT STATUS: ☐ YES: ☐ NO:

MECHANISMS OF ACTION:	CONTRAINDICATIONS:	SAFETY & ANTIDOTE:
DOSAGE & ROUTE:	SIDE EFFECTS: (ADVERSE REACTION)	THERAPEUPIC USE:

PATIENT EDUCATION:	NURSING ASSESSMENTS / INTERVENTIONS:

NOTE:

GENERIC NAME:	DRUG NAME:
DRUG CLASS:	HIGH ALERT STATUS: ☐ YES: ☐ NO:

MECHANISMS OF ACTION:	CONTRAINDICATIONS:	SAFETY & ANTIDOTE:
DOSAGE & ROUTE:	SIDE EFFECTS: (ADVERSE REACTION)	THERAPEUPIC USE:

PATIENT EDUCATION:	NURSING ASSESSMENTS / INTERVENTIONS:

NOTE:

GENERIC NAME:	DRUG NAME:
DRUG CLASS:	HIGH ALERT STATUS: ☐ YES: ☐ NO:

MECHANISMS OF ACTION:	CONTRAINDICATIONS:	SAFETY & ANTIDOTE:
DOSAGE & ROUTE:	SIDE EFFECTS: (ADVERSE REACTION)	THERAPEUPIC USE:

PATIENT EDUCATION:	NURSING ASSESSMENTS / INTERVENTIONS:

NOTE:

GENERIC NAME:

DRUG NAME:

DRUG CLASS:

HIGH ALERT STATUS: ☐ YES: ☐ NO:

MECHANISMS OF ACTION:

CONTRAINDICATIONS:

SAFETY & ANTIDOTE:

DOSAGE & ROUTE:

SIDE EFFECTS:
(ADVERSE REACTION)

THERAPEUPIC USE:

PATIENT EDUCATION:

NURSING ASSESSMENTS / INTERVENTIONS:

NOTE:

GENERIC NAME:	DRUG NAME:
DRUG CLASS:	HIGH ALERT STATUS: ☐ YES: ☐ NO:

MECHANISMS OF ACTION:	CONTRAINDICATIONS:	SAFETY & ANTIDOTE:
DOSAGE & ROUTE:	SIDE EFFECTS: (ADVERSE REACTION)	THERAPEUPIC USE:

PATIENT EDUCATION:	NURSING ASSESSMENTS / INTERVENTIONS:

NOTE:

GENERIC NAME:	DRUG NAME:
DRUG CLASS:	HIGH ALERT STATUS: ☐ YES: ☐ NO:

MECHANISMS OF ACTION:	CONTRAINDICATIONS:	SAFETY & ANTIDOTE:
DOSAGE & ROUTE:	SIDE EFFECTS: (ADVERSE REACTION)	THERAPEUPIC USE:

PATIENT EDUCATION:	NURSING ASSESSMENTS / INTERVENTIONS:

NOTE:

GENERIC NAME:	DRUG NAME:
DRUG CLASS:	HIGH ALERT STATUS: ☐ YES: ☐ NO:

MECHANISMS OF ACTION:	CONTRAINDICATIONS:	SAFETY & ANTIDOTE:
DOSAGE & ROUTE:	SIDE EFFECTS: (ADVERSE REACTION)	THERAPEUPIC USE:

PATIENT EDUCATION:	NURSING ASSESSMENTS / INTERVENTIONS:

NOTE:

GENERIC NAME:	DRUG NAME:
DRUG CLASS:	HIGH ALERT STATUS: ☐ YES: ☐ NO:

MECHANISMS OF ACTION:	CONTRAINDICATIONS:	SAFETY & ANTIDOTE:
DOSAGE & ROUTE:	SIDE EFFECTS: (ADVERSE REACTION)	THERAPEUPIC USE:

PATIENT EDUCATION:	NURSING ASSESSMENTS / INTERVENTIONS:

NOTE:

GENERIC NAME:	DRUG NAME:
DRUG CLASS:	HIGH ALERT STATUS: ☐ YES: ☐ NO:

MECHANISMS OF ACTION:	CONTRAINDICATIONS:	SAFETY & ANTIDOTE:
DOSAGE & ROUTE:	SIDE EFFECTS: (ADVERSE REACTION)	THERAPEUPIC USE:

PATIENT EDUCATION:	NURSING ASSESSMENTS / INTERVENTIONS:

NOTE:

GENERIC NAME:	DRUG NAME:
DRUG CLASS:	HIGH ALERT STATUS: ☐ YES: ☐ NO:

MECHANISMS OF ACTION:	CONTRAINDICATIONS:	SAFETY & ANTIDOTE:
DOSAGE & ROUTE:	SIDE EFFECTS: (ADVERSE REACTION)	THERAPEUPIC USE:

PATIENT EDUCATION:	NURSING ASSESSMENTS / INTERVENTIONS:

NOTE:

GENERIC NAME:	DRUG NAME:
DRUG CLASS:	HIGH ALERT STATUS: ☐ YES: ☐ NO:

MECHANISMS OF ACTION:	CONTRAINDICATIONS:	SAFETY & ANTIDOTE:
DOSAGE & ROUTE:	SIDE EFFECTS: (ADVERSE REACTION)	THERAPEUPIC USE:

PATIENT EDUCATION:	NURSING ASSESSMENTS / INTERVENTIONS:

NOTE:

GENERIC NAME:	DRUG NAME:
DRUG CLASS:	HIGH ALERT STATUS: ☐ YES: ☐ NO:

MECHANISMS OF ACTION:	CONTRAINDICATIONS:	SAFETY & ANTIDOTE:
DOSAGE & ROUTE:	SIDE EFFECTS: (ADVERSE REACTION)	THERAPEUPIC USE:

PATIENT EDUCATION:	NURSING ASSESSMENTS / INTERVENTIONS:

NOTE:

GENERIC NAME:	DRUG NAME:
DRUG CLASS:	HIGH ALERT STATUS: ☐ YES: ☐ NO:

MECHANISMS OF ACTION:	CONTRAINDICATIONS:	SAFETY & ANTIDOTE:
DOSAGE & ROUTE:	SIDE EFFECTS: (ADVERSE REACTION)	THERAPEUPIC USE:

PATIENT EDUCATION:	NURSING ASSESSMENTS / INTERVENTIONS:

NOTE:

GENERIC NAME:	DRUG NAME:
DRUG CLASS:	HIGH ALERT STATUS: ☐ YES: ☐ NO:

MECHANISMS OF ACTION:	CONTRAINDICATIONS:	SAFETY & ANTIDOTE:
DOSAGE & ROUTE:	SIDE EFFECTS: (ADVERSE REACTION)	THERAPEUPIC USE:

PATIENT EDUCATION:	NURSING ASSESSMENTS / INTERVENTIONS:

NOTE:

GENERIC NAME:	DRUG NAME:
DRUG CLASS:	HIGH ALERT STATUS: ☐ YES: ☐ NO:

MECHANISMS OF ACTION:	CONTRAINDICATIONS:	SAFETY & ANTIDOTE:
DOSAGE & ROUTE:	SIDE EFFECTS: (ADVERSE REACTION)	THERAPEUPIC USE:

PATIENT EDUCATION:	NURSING ASSESSMENTS / INTERVENTIONS:

NOTE:

GENERIC NAME:	DRUG NAME:
DRUG CLASS:	HIGH ALERT STATUS: ☐ YES: ☐ NO:

MECHANISMS OF ACTION:	CONTRAINDICATIONS:	SAFETY & ANTIDOTE:
DOSAGE & ROUTE:	SIDE EFFECTS: (ADVERSE REACTION)	THERAPEUPIC USE:

PATIENT EDUCATION:	NURSING ASSESSMENTS / INTERVENTIONS:

NOTE:

GENERIC NAME:	DRUG NAME:
DRUG CLASS:	HIGH ALERT STATUS: ☐ YES: ☐ NO:

MECHANISMS OF ACTION:	CONTRAINDICATIONS:	SAFETY & ANTIDOTE:
DOSAGE & ROUTE:	SIDE EFFECTS: (ADVERSE REACTION)	THERAPEUPIC USE:

PATIENT EDUCATION:	NURSING ASSESSMENTS / INTERVENTIONS:

NOTE:

GENERIC NAME:	DRUG NAME:
DRUG CLASS:	HIGH ALERT STATUS: ☐ YES: ☐ NO:

MECHANISMS OF ACTION:	CONTRAINDICATIONS:	SAFETY & ANTIDOTE:
DOSAGE & ROUTE:	SIDE EFFECTS: (ADVERSE REACTION)	THERAPEUPIC USE:

PATIENT EDUCATION:	NURSING ASSESSMENTS / INTERVENTIONS:

NOTE:

GENERIC NAME:	DRUG NAME:
DRUG CLASS:	HIGH ALERT STATUS: ☐ YES: ☐ NO:

MECHANISMS OF ACTION:	CONTRAINDICATIONS:	SAFETY & ANTIDOTE:
DOSAGE & ROUTE:	SIDE EFFECTS: (ADVERSE REACTION)	THERAPEUPIC USE:

PATIENT EDUCATION:	NURSING ASSESSMENTS / INTERVENTIONS:

NOTE:

GENERIC NAME:	DRUG NAME:
DRUG CLASS:	HIGH ALERT STATUS: ☐ YES: ☐ NO:

MECHANISMS OF ACTION:	CONTRAINDICATIONS:	SAFETY & ANTIDOTE:
DOSAGE & ROUTE:	SIDE EFFECTS: (ADVERSE REACTION)	THERAPEUPIC USE:

PATIENT EDUCATION:	NURSING ASSESSMENTS / INTERVENTIONS:

NOTE:

NURSING PHARMACOLOGY MEDICATION SHEET

GENERIC NAME:	DRUG NAME:
DRUG CLASS:	HIGH ALERT STATUS: ☐ YES: ☐ NO:

MECHANISMS OF ACTION:	CONTRAINDICATIONS:	SAFETY & ANTIDOTE:
DOSAGE & ROUTE:	SIDE EFFECTS: (ADVERSE REACTION)	THERAPEUPIC USE:

PATIENT EDUCATION:	NURSING ASSESSMENTS / INTERVENTIONS:

NOTE:

GENERIC NAME:	DRUG NAME:
DRUG CLASS:	HIGH ALERT STATUS: ☐ YES: ☐ NO:

MECHANISMS OF ACTION:	CONTRAINDICATIONS:	SAFETY & ANTIDOTE:
DOSAGE & ROUTE:	SIDE EFFECTS: (ADVERSE REACTION)	THERAPEUPIC USE:

PATIENT EDUCATION:	NURSING ASSESSMENTS / INTERVENTIONS:

NOTE:

GENERIC NAME:	DRUG NAME:
DRUG CLASS:	HIGH ALERT STATUS: ☐ YES: ☐ NO:

MECHANISMS OF ACTION:	CONTRAINDICATIONS:	SAFETY & ANTIDOTE:
DOSAGE & ROUTE:	SIDE EFFECTS: (ADVERSE REACTION)	THERAPEUPIC USE:

PATIENT EDUCATION:	NURSING ASSESSMENTS / INTERVENTIONS:

NOTE:

GENERIC NAME:	DRUG NAME:
DRUG CLASS:	HIGH ALERT STATUS: ☐ YES: ☐ NO:

MECHANISMS OF ACTION:	CONTRAINDICATIONS:	SAFETY & ANTIDOTE:
DOSAGE & ROUTE:	SIDE EFFECTS: (ADVERSE REACTION)	THERAPEUPIC USE:

PATIENT EDUCATION:	NURSING ASSESSMENTS / INTERVENTIONS:

NOTE:

GENERIC NAME:	DRUG NAME:
DRUG CLASS:	HIGH ALERT STATUS: ☐ YES: ☐ NO:

MECHANISMS OF ACTION:	CONTRAINDICATIONS:	SAFETY & ANTIDOTE:
DOSAGE & ROUTE:	SIDE EFFECTS: (ADVERSE REACTION)	THERAPEUPIC USE:

PATIENT EDUCATION:	NURSING ASSESSMENTS / INTERVENTIONS:

NOTE:

GENERIC NAME:	DRUG NAME:
DRUG CLASS:	HIGH ALERT STATUS: ☐ YES: ☐ NO:

MECHANISMS OF ACTION:	CONTRAINDICATIONS:	SAFETY & ANTIDOTE:
DOSAGE & ROUTE:	SIDE EFFECTS: (ADVERSE REACTION)	THERAPEUPIC USE:

PATIENT EDUCATION:	NURSING ASSESSMENTS / INTERVENTIONS:

NOTE:

GENERIC NAME:

DRUG NAME:

DRUG CLASS:

HIGH ALERT STATUS: ☐ YES: ☐ NO:

MECHANISMS OF ACTION:

CONTRAINDICATIONS:

SAFETY & ANTIDOTE:

DOSAGE & ROUTE:

SIDE EFFECTS:
(ADVERSE REACTION)

THERAPEUPIC USE:

PATIENT EDUCATION:

NURSING ASSESSMENTS / INTERVENTIONS:

NOTE:

GENERIC NAME:	DRUG NAME:
DRUG CLASS:	HIGH ALERT STATUS: ☐ YES: ☐ NO:

MECHANISMS OF ACTION:	CONTRAINDICATIONS:	SAFETY & ANTIDOTE:
DOSAGE & ROUTE:	SIDE EFFECTS: (ADVERSE REACTION)	THERAPEUPIC USE:

PATIENT EDUCATION:	NURSING ASSESSMENTS / INTERVENTIONS:

NOTE:

GENERIC NAME:	DRUG NAME:
DRUG CLASS:	HIGH ALERT STATUS: ☐ YES: ☐ NO:

MECHANISMS OF ACTION:	CONTRAINDICATIONS:	SAFETY & ANTIDOTE:
DOSAGE & ROUTE:	SIDE EFFECTS: (ADVERSE REACTION)	THERAPEUPIC USE:

PATIENT EDUCATION:	NURSING ASSESSMENTS / INTERVENTIONS:

NOTE:

Thank you so much

Check Out Our Other Books.
www.udesme.com

Published by Udesme, a pen name for Rita Udesi Johnson, United Kingdom.

ISBN 978-1-917602-37-2

Made in the USA
Monee, IL
04 November 2026

67384405R00069